VEGETARIAN TYPE 2 DIABETES COOKBOOK FOR BEGINNERS

Your 30-Day Vegetarian Roadmap to Managing Type 2 Diabetes with Easy Recipes

T. John

COPYRIGHT PAGE

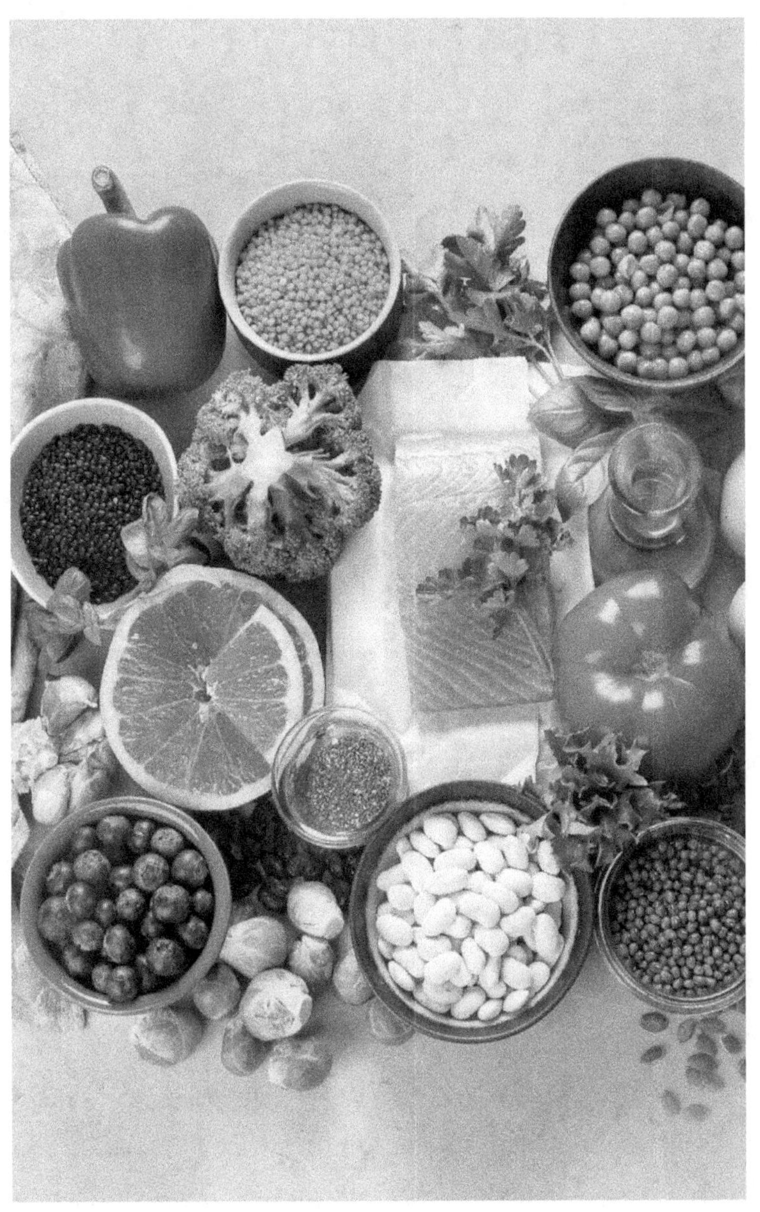

TABLE OF CONTENTS

Chapter 5: Snacks and Appetizers 82

INTRODUCTION

Living with type 2 diabetes can feel like navigating a complex maze. Blood sugar spikes, medication routines, and dietary choices all become intertwined, making the path to optimal health appear shrouded in confusion. But fear not, fellow traveler! By understanding the link between diabetes, nutrition, and the potential of a vegetarian diet, you can transform this maze into a vibrant garden of possibilities.

Type 2 Diabetes: A Story of Insulin Resistance

Imagine your body as a bustling city, and insulin as the traffic warden, ensuring glucose (sugar), the city's fuel, reaches its designated buildings (cells) for energy production. In type 2 diabetes, this system malfunctions. The traffic warden (insulin) becomes sluggish, and the buildings (cells) grow less receptive to the sugar flowing through the bloodstream. This gridlock leads to high blood sugar levels, the hallmark of diabetes.

Nutrition: The Master Key to Unlocking Control

Now, let's talk diet, the master key to unlocking glycemic control. A balanced, nutritious diet is the cornerstone of effective diabetes management. But with so much conflicting information, where do we begin?

Enter the Vegetarian Stage: A Symphony of Plant-Based Goodness

A well-planned vegetarian diet, encompassing lacto-ovo (including eggs and dairy) or vegan (excluding all animal products) variations, can be a powerful tool in the fight against diabetes. Here's why:

1. **Fiber Fiesta**: Vegetables, fruits, legumes and whole grains are fiber superstars, slowing down sugar absorption and preventing blood sugar spikes. Think of fiber as the city's detour lanes, easing traffic flow and preventing congestion.

2. **Weight-Wise Warriors**: Vegetarian diets tend to be naturally lower in calorie density and unhealthy fats, promoting weight management, a crucial factor in

diabetes control. Imagine a slimmer traffic warden navigating the city with greater agility!

3. **Antioxidant Allure**: Plant-based foods are bursting with antioxidants, those microscopic shields protecting your cells from harmful free radicals. Think of antioxidants as the city's sanitation workers, keeping everything clean and running smoothly.

4. **Vitamin Bounty**: Vegetarian diets are rich in essential vitamins and minerals, like magnesium and vitamin B12, which play a crucial role in insulin function and overall health. Imagine these as the city's well-maintained infrastructure, ensuring smooth operation of all systems.

Beyond the Benefits: Addressing Concerns

While a vegetarian diet offers a wealth of advantages, some concerns linger. Protein intake, iron deficiency, and vitamin B12 are common questions. But fret not!

1. **Protein Powerhouse**: Legumes, lentils, nuts, seeds, and dairy products (in lacto-ovo diets) provide ample protein, making it easy to meet your daily needs.

Imagine a diverse range of food trucks lining the city streets, offering a variety of protein-rich delicacies.

2. **Ironclad Defense**: Leafy greens, quinoa, beans, and lentils are iron champions, readily available in the plant kingdom. Plus, vitamin C-rich fruits and vegetables enhance iron absorption. Imagine these as iron supplement shops strategically located throughout the city.

3. **B12 Bonanza**: Fortified plant milks, nutritional yeast, and certain mushrooms come to the rescue, ensuring adequate B12 intake. Consider these your B12 bakeries, spreading goodness throughout the city.

Remember, a well-planned vegetarian diet, along with regular exercise and proper medical guidance, can be a game-changer in diabetes management. So, embrace the vibrant world of plant-based possibilities, and watch your diabetes maze transform into a flourishing garden of health and well-being!

Chapter 1: 30 Day Meal Plan

Week 1:

Day 1:

- Breakfast: Avocado and Tomato Breakfast Wrap
- Lunch: Lentil and Vegetable Soup
- Dinner: Cauliflower and Broccoli Bake
- Snack: Guacamole with Veggie Sticks
- Dessert: Berry and Chia Seed Popsicles

Day 2:

- Breakfast: Quinoa Porridge with Berries
- Lunch: Quinoa and Black Bean Salad
- Dinner: Portobello Mushroom Steaks
- Snack: Edamame Hummus with Whole Grain Crackers
- Dessert: Dark Chocolate-Dipped Strawberries

Day 3:

- Breakfast: Spinach and Feta Omelette
- Lunch: Chickpea and Spinach Stuffed Bell Peppers

- Dinner: Ratatouille with Quinoa
- Snack: Roasted Chickpeas with Cumin
- Dessert: Baked Apple with Cinnamon

Day 4:

- Breakfast: Chia Seed Pudding with Almond Milk
- Lunch: Grilled Eggplant and Hummus Wrap
- Dinner: Spaghetti Squash Primavera
- Snack: Greek Yogurt and Berry Parfait
- Dessert: Avocado Chocolate Mousse

Day 5:

- Breakfast: Greek Yogurt Parfait with Nuts
- Lunch: Zucchini Noodles with Pesto
- Dinner: Thai Red Curry with Tofu
- Snack: Sliced Apple with Almond Butter
- Dessert: Coconut and Berry Sorbet

Day 6:

- Breakfast: Veggie-loaded Tofu Scramble
- Lunch: Brown Rice and Vegetable Stir-Fry
- Dinner: Eggplant Parmesan

- Snack: Veggie Spring Rolls with Peanut Sauce
- Dessert: Pumpkin Pie Smoothie

Day 7:

- Breakfast: Whole Grain Pancakes with Berry Compote
- Lunch: Caprese Salad with Avocado
- Dinner: Stuffed Acorn Squash with Wild Rice
- Snack: Caprese Skewers with Balsamic Glaze
- Dessert: Almond Flour Blueberry Muffins

Week 2:

Day 8:

- Breakfast: Mushroom and Spinach Breakfast Casserole
- Lunch: Sweet Potato and Chickpea Curry
- Dinner: Cabbage and Lentil Casserole
- Snack: Almond and Coconut Energy Bites
- Dessert: Banana and Walnut Bread

Day 9:

- Breakfast: Oatmeal with Walnuts and Apples

- Lunch: Spinach and Quinoa Stuffed Tomatoes
- Dinner: Quinoa-stuffed Bell Peppers
- Snack: Stuffed Mini Bell Peppers with Herbed Cream Cheese
- Dessert: Greek Yogurt and Honey Parfait

Day 10:

- Breakfast: Broccoli and Cheese Breakfast Muffins
- Lunch: Cucumber and Avocado Sushi Rolls
- Dinner: Sweet Potato and Black Bean Enchiladas
- Snack: Sweet Potato Fries with Avocado Dip
- Dessert: Mango and Coconut Chia Pudding

Day 11:

- Breakfast: Banana and Almond Butter Smoothie Bowl
- Lunch: Mediterranean Chickpea Salad
- Dinner: Mushroom and Spinach Lasagna
- Snack: Cucumber Cups with Tzatziki
- Dessert: Raspberry Oat Bars

Day 12:

- Breakfast: Blueberry Almond Baked Oatmeal
- Lunch: Butternut Squash and Kale Salad
- Dinner: Teriyaki Tofu Stir-Fry
- Snack: Avocado and Black Bean Salsa
- Dessert: Quinoa Chocolate Chip Cookies

Day 13:

- Breakfast: Veggie Breakfast Quesadilla
- Lunch: Black Bean and Corn Quesadilla
- Dinner: Lentil and Vegetable Curry
- Snack: Tomato Basil Bruschetta
- Dessert: Pistachio and Cranberry Energy Balls

Day 14:

- Breakfast: Coconut Yogurt Parfait with Granola
- Lunch: Mushroom and Lentil Lettuce Wraps
- Dinner: Spinach and Ricotta Stuffed Shells
- Snack: Mixed Nuts and Seeds Trail Mix
- Dessert: Lemon Poppy Seed Cake

Week 3:

Day 15:

- Breakfast: Coconut Yogurt Parfait with Granola
- Lunch: Greek Salad with Tofu Feta
- Dinner: Vegan Chili with Kidney Beans
- Snack: Roasted Red Pepper Hummus with Pita Chips
- Dessert: Vegan Chocolate Avocado Cake

Day 16:

- Breakfast: Avocado and Tomato Breakfast Wrap
- Lunch: Lentil and Vegetable Soup
- Dinner: Cauliflower and Broccoli Bake
- Snack: Guacamole with Veggie Sticks
- Dessert: Berry and Chia Seed Popsicles

Day 17:

- Breakfast: Quinoa Porridge with Berries
- Lunch: Quinoa and Black Bean Salad
- Dinner: Portobello Mushroom Steaks
- Snack: Edamame Hummus with Whole Grain Crackers
- Dessert: Dark Chocolate-Dipped Strawberries

Day 18:

- Breakfast: Spinach and Feta Omelette
- Lunch: Chickpea and Spinach Stuffed Bell Peppers
- Dinner: Ratatouille with Quinoa
- Snack: Roasted Chickpeas with Cumin
- Dessert: Baked Apple with Cinnamon

Day 19:

- Breakfast: Chia Seed Pudding with Almond Milk
- Lunch: Grilled Eggplant and Hummus Wrap
- Dinner: Spaghetti Squash Primavera
- Snack: Greek Yogurt and Berry Parfait
- Dessert: Avocado Chocolate Mousse

Day 20:

- Breakfast: Greek Yogurt Parfait with Nuts
- Lunch: Zucchini Noodles with Pesto
- Dinner: Thai Red Curry with Tofu
- Snack: Sliced Apple with Almond Butter
- Dessert: Coconut and Berry Sorbet

Day 21:

- Breakfast: Veggie-loaded Tofu Scramble
- Lunch: Brown Rice and Vegetable Stir-Fry
- Dinner: Eggplant Parmesan
- Snack: Veggie Spring Rolls with Peanut Sauce
- Dessert: Pumpkin Pie Smoothie

Week 4:

Day 22:

- Breakfast: Whole Grain Pancakes with Berry Compote
- Lunch: Caprese Salad with Avocado
- Dinner: Stuffed Acorn Squash with Wild Rice
- Snack: Caprese Skewers with Balsamic Glaze
- Dessert: Almond Flour Blueberry Muffins

Day 23:

- Breakfast: Mushroom and Spinach Breakfast Casserole
- Lunch: Sweet Potato and Chickpea Curry
- Dinner: Cabbage and Lentil Casserole
- Snack: Almond and Coconut Energy Bites

- Dessert: Banana and Walnut Bread

Day 24:

- Breakfast: Oatmeal with Walnuts and Apples
- Lunch: Spinach and Quinoa Stuffed Tomatoes
- Dinner: Quinoa-stuffed Bell Peppers
- Snack: Stuffed Mini Bell Peppers with Herbed Cream Cheese
- Dessert: Greek Yogurt and Honey Parfait

Day 25:

- Breakfast: Broccoli and Cheese Breakfast Muffins
- Lunch: Cucumber and Avocado Sushi Rolls
- Dinner: Sweet Potato and Black Bean Enchiladas
- Snack: Sweet Potato Fries with Avocado Dip
- Dessert: Mango and Coconut Chia Pudding

Day 26:

- Breakfast: Banana and Almond Butter Smoothie Bowl
- Lunch: Mediterranean Chickpea Salad
- Dinner: Mushroom and Spinach Lasagna

- Snack: Cucumber Cups with Tzatziki
- Dessert: Raspberry Oat Bars

Day 27:

- Breakfast: Blueberry Almond Baked Oatmeal
- Lunch: Butternut Squash and Kale Salad
- Dinner: Teriyaki Tofu Stir-Fry
- Snack: Avocado and Black Bean Salsa
- Dessert: Quinoa Chocolate Chip Cookies

Day 28:

- Breakfast: Veggie Breakfast Quesadilla
- Lunch: Black Bean and Corn Quesadilla
- Dinner: Lentil and Vegetable Curry
- Snack: Tomato Basil Bruschetta
- Dessert: Pistachio and Cranberry Energy Balls

Day 29:

- Breakfast: Coconut Yogurt Parfait with Granola
- Lunch: Mushroom and Lentil Lettuce Wraps
- Dinner: Spinach and Ricotta Stuffed Shells
- Snack: Mixed Nuts and Seeds Trail Mix

- Dessert: Lemon Poppy Seed Cake

Day 30:

- Breakfast: Coconut Yogurt Parfait with Granola

- Lunch: Greek Salad with Tofu Feta

- Dinner: Vegan Chili with Kidney Beans

- Snack: Roasted Red Pepper Hummus with Pita Chips

- Dessert: Vegan Chocolate Avocado Cake

Chapter 2: Breakfast Recipes

In this chapter, we've curated breakfast recipes that are not only delicious but also tailored for individuals managing type 2 diabetes. Each recipe is crafted with a variety of nutrient-rich ingredients to ensure a balanced and satisfying start to your day.

Avocado and Tomato Breakfast Wrap

Ingredients:

- 1 whole-grain tortilla
- 1 ripe avocado, sliced
- 1 medium tomato, diced
- 1 tablespoon olive oil
- Salt and pepper to taste

Instructions:

1. Heat the tortilla in a pan.
2. Spread sliced avocado evenly.
3. Add diced tomatoes.

4. Drizzle with olive oil.

5. Season with salt and pepper.

6. Roll up and enjoy!

Nutrition Information:

- Calories: 300

- Protein: 6g

- Carbohydrates: 25g

- Fat: 20g

- Fiber: 8g

- Sugar: 2g

- Portion Size: 1 wrap

Quinoa Porridge with Berries

Ingredients:

- 1/2 cup quinoa, rinsed

- 1 cup almond milk

- 1/2 cup mixed berries

- 1 tablespoon honey

- 1/4 teaspoon vanilla extract

Instructions:

1. Cook quinoa in almond milk.
2. Add berries, honey, and vanilla.
3. Stir and simmer until creamy.
4. Serve warm.

Nutrition Information:

- Calories: 280
- Protein: 7g
- Carbohydrates: 45g
- Fat: 6g
- Fiber: 6g
- Sugar: 8g
- Portion Size: 1 cup

Spinach and Feta Omelette

Ingredients:

- 2 eggs, beaten
- 1 cup fresh spinach
- 1/4 cup feta cheese, crumbled
- Salt and pepper to taste

Instructions:

1. Sauté spinach until wilted.
2. Pour beaten eggs over spinach.
3. Add feta, salt, and pepper.
4. Cook until eggs set.
5. Fold and serve.

Nutrition Information:

- Calories: 220
- Protein: 16g
- Carbohydrates: 3g
- Fat: 16g
- Fiber: 1g
- Sugar: 1g
- Portion Size: 1 omelette

Chia Seed Pudding with Almond Milk

Ingredients:

- 2 tablespoons chia seeds
- 1 cup unsweetened almond milk
- 1 tablespoon maple syrup
- 1/2 teaspoon vanilla extract

- Fresh berries for topping

Instructions:

1. Mix chia seeds, almond milk, maple syrup, and vanilla.
2. Refrigerate for at least 4 hours or overnight.
3. Top with fresh berries before serving.

Nutrition Information:

- Calories: 180
- Protein: 5g
- Carbohydrates: 20g
- Fat: 10g
- Fiber: 8g
- Sugar: 6g
- Portion Size: 1 cup

Greek Yogurt Parfait with Nuts

Ingredients:

- 1 cup Greek yogurt
- 1/2 cup granola
- 1/4 cup mixed nuts (almonds, walnuts)

- 1 tablespoon honey

Instructions:

1. Layer Greek yogurt and granola.

2. Add a layer of mixed nuts.

3. Drizzle with honey.

4. Repeat layers.

5. Enjoy!

Nutrition Information:

- Calories: 320

- Protein: 18g

- Carbohydrates: 30g

- Fat: 15g

- Fiber: 4g

- Sugar: 12g

- Portion Size: 1 serving

Veggie-loaded Tofu Scramble

Ingredients:

- 1/2 cup firm tofu, crumbled

- 1/2 cup bell peppers, diced

- 1/4 cup red onion, chopped

- 1 cup spinach

- 1 tablespoon olive oil

- Salt and pepper to taste

Instructions:

1. Sauté bell peppers and onion in olive oil.

2. Add crumbled tofu.

3. Stir in spinach until wilted.

4. Season with salt and pepper.

5. Serve warm.

Nutrition Information:

- Calories: 220

- Protein: 15g

- Carbohydrates: 10g

- Fat: 14g

- Fiber: 3g

- Sugar: 2g

- Portion Size: 1 serving

Whole Grain Pancakes with Berry Compote

Ingredients:

- 1 cup whole grain pancake mix
- 3/4 cup water
- 1 cup mixed berries
- 2 tablespoons maple syrup

Instructions:

1. Prepare pancake mix with water.
2. Cook pancakes on a griddle.
3. In a saucepan, simmer berries and syrup.
4. Top pancakes with berry compote.

Nutrition Information:

- Calories: 280
- Protein: 8g
- Carbohydrates: 55g
- Fat: 3g
- Fiber: 7g
- Sugar: 12g
- Portion Size: 2 pancakes with compote

Sweet Potato and Black Bean Breakfast Burrito

Ingredients:

- 1 whole-grain tortilla
- 1/2 cup sweet potatoes, cooked and mashed
- 1/4 cup black beans, drained and rinsed
- 2 eggs, scrambled
- Salsa for topping

Instructions:

1. Spread mashed sweet potatoes on a tortilla.
2. Add black beans and scrambled eggs.
3. Roll up and top with salsa.
4. Enjoy!

Nutrition Information:

- Calories: 310
- Protein: 15g
- Carbohydrates: 40g
- Fat: 10g
- Fiber: 8g
- Sugar: 2g

- Portion Size: 1 burrito

Mushroom and Spinach Breakfast Casserole

Ingredients:

- 1 cup mushrooms, sliced
- 1 cup fresh spinach
- 6 eggs, beaten
- 1/2 cup milk
- 1/2 cup feta cheese, crumbled

Instructions:

1. Sauté mushrooms until golden.
2. Add spinach and cook until wilted.
3. Whisk eggs and milk together.
4. Mix in sautéed mushrooms and spinach.
5. Pour into a baking dish, top with feta.
6. Bake until eggs are set.

Nutrition Information:

- Calories: 250

- Protein: 17g

- Carbohydrates: 6g

- Fat: 18g

- Fiber: 2g

- Sugar: 3g

- Portion Size: 1 serving

Oatmeal with Walnuts and Apples

Ingredients:

- 1/2 cup old-fashioned oats

- 1 cup water

- 1/2 apple, diced

- 1 tablespoon chopped walnuts

- 1 teaspoon cinnamon

Instructions:

1. Cook oats in water until creamy.

2. Stir in diced apples, walnuts, and cinnamon.

3. Simmer until apples are tender.

4. Serve warm.

Nutrition Information:

- Calories: 220
- Protein: 6g
- Carbohydrates: 35g
- Fat: 8g
- Fiber: 6g
- Sugar: 10g
- Portion Size: 1 serving

Broccoli and Cheese Breakfast Muffins

Ingredients:

- 2 cups broccoli, chopped
- 1/2 cup cheddar cheese, shredded
- 6 eggs, beaten
- Salt and pepper to taste

Instructions:

1. Steam broccoli until tender.
2. Mix broccoli with beaten eggs, cheese, salt, and pepper.

3. Pour into muffin cups.

4. Bake until set.

Nutrition Information:

- Calories: 180

- Protein: 14g

- Carbohydrates: 5g

- Fat: 12g

- Fiber: 2g

- Sugar: 1g

- Portion Size: 2 muffins

Banana and Almond Butter Smoothie Bowl

Ingredients:

- 2 ripe bananas

- 2 tablespoons almond butter

- 1 cup almond milk

- 1/2 cup granola

- Sliced almonds for topping

Instructions:

1. Blend bananas, almond butter, and almond milk.
2. Pour into a bowl.
3. Top with granola and sliced almonds.

Nutrition Information:

- Calories: 320
- Protein: 8g
- Carbohydrates: 45g
- Fat: 15g
- Fiber: 7g
- Sugar: 18g
- Portion Size: 1 bowl

Blueberry Almond Baked Oatmeal

Ingredients:

- 1 cup old-fashioned oats
- 1/2 cup almond milk
- 1/4 cup maple syrup
- 1/2 cup blueberries
- 1/4 cup chopped almonds
- 1 teaspoon vanilla extract

Instructions:

1. Mix oats, almond milk, maple syrup, blueberries, almonds, and vanilla.
2. Pour into a baking dish.
3. Bake until golden and set.
4. Serve warm.

Nutrition Information:

- Calories: 260
- Protein: 7g
- Carbohydrates: 40g
- Fat: 8g
- Fiber: 6g
- Sugar: 16g
- Portion Size: 1 serving

Veggie Breakfast Quesadilla

Ingredients:

- 1 whole-grain tortilla
- 1/2 cup black beans, mashed
- 1/4 cup bell peppers, diced
- 1/4 cup red onion, sliced

- 1/2 cup spinach
- 1/4 cup shredded cheese

Instructions:

1. Spread mashed black beans on a tortilla.
2. Add diced bell peppers, red onion, and spinach.
3. Sprinkle with shredded cheese.
4. Top with another tortilla and cook until cheese melts.
5. Slice and enjoy!

Nutrition Information:

- Calories: 290
- Protein: 15g
- Carbohydrates: 45g
- Fat: 8g
- Fiber: 10g
- Sugar: 2g
- Portion Size: 1 quesadilla

Coconut Yogurt Parfait with Granola

Ingredients:

- 1 cup coconut yogurt

- 1/2 cup granola
- 1/4 cup shredded coconut
- Mixed berries for topping

Instructions:

1. Layer coconut yogurt and granola.
2. Add a layer of shredded coconut.
3. Top with mixed berries.
4. Repeat layers.
5. Enjoy!

Nutrition Information:

- Calories: 330
- Protein: 8g
- Carbohydrates: 45g
- Fat: 15g
- Fiber: 6g
- Sugar: 18g
- Portion Size: 1 serving

Chapter 3: Lunch Recipes

In this chapter, we've crafted flavorful and diabetes-friendly vegetarian lunch recipes that not only tantalize your taste buds but also contribute to a balanced and healthy lifestyle. Each recipe is carefully designed to offer a variety of nutrients while keeping a check on calories, protein, carbohydrates, fats, fiber, and sugar.

Lentil and Vegetable Soup

Ingredients:

- 1 cup green lentils, rinsed
- 4 cups vegetable broth
- 1 onion, diced
- 2 carrots, chopped
- 2 celery stalks, sliced
- 1 can diced tomatoes
- 2 cloves garlic, minced
- 1 teaspoon cumin
- 1 teaspoon paprika
- Salt and pepper to taste

Instructions:

1. In a large pot, sauté onions and garlic until fragrant.
2. Add lentils, vegetable broth, carrots, celery, diced tomatoes, cumin, paprika, salt, and pepper.
3. Bring to a boil, then simmer until lentils are tender.
4. Adjust seasoning and serve hot.

Nutrition Information:

- Calories: 250
- Protein: 15g
- Carbohydrates: 40g
- Fat: 2g
- Fiber: 12g
- Sugar: 5g
- Portion Size: 1 cup

Quinoa and Black Bean Salad

Ingredients:

- 1 cup quinoa, cooked
- 1 can black beans, drained and rinsed
- 1 cup cherry tomatoes, halved
- 1 cucumber, diced

- 1/4 cup red onion, finely chopped
- 1/4 cup fresh cilantro, chopped
- Juice of 1 lime
- 2 tablespoons olive oil
- Salt and pepper to taste

Instructions:

1. In a large bowl, combine quinoa, black beans, cherry tomatoes, cucumber, red onion, and cilantro.
2. In a small bowl, whisk together lime juice, olive oil, salt, and pepper.
3. Pour dressing over the salad and toss gently.
4. Chill before serving.

Nutrition Information:

- Calories: 320
- Protein: 12g
- Carbohydrates: 50g
- Fat: 8g
- Fiber: 10g
- Sugar: 3g
- Portion Size: 1 cup

Chickpea and Spinach Stuffed Bell Peppers

Ingredients:

- 4 bell peppers, halved and seeds removed
- 1 can chickpeas, drained and mashed
- 2 cups spinach, chopped
- 1 cup cooked quinoa
- 1/2 cup feta cheese, crumbled
- 1 teaspoon cumin
- 1/2 teaspoon garlic powder
- Salt and pepper to taste

Instructions:

1. Preheat the oven to 375°F (190°C).
2. In a bowl, mix mashed chickpeas, spinach, cooked quinoa, feta, cumin, garlic powder, salt, and pepper.
3. Stuff each bell pepper half with the mixture.
4. Bake for 25-30 minutes until peppers are tender.

Nutrition Information:

- Calories: 180
- Protein: 8g

- Carbohydrates: 30g

- Fat: 4g

- Fiber: 8g

- Sugar: 5g

- Portion Size: 1 stuffed pepper half

Grilled Eggplant and Hummus Wrap

Ingredients:

- 1 large eggplant, sliced

- 4 whole-grain wraps

- 1 cup hummus

- 1 cup cherry tomatoes, sliced

- 1/2 cup cucumber, julienned

- Fresh mint leaves

- Salt and pepper to taste

Instructions:

1. Grill eggplant slices until tender.

2. Spread hummus on each wrap.

3. Place grilled eggplant, cherry tomatoes, cucumber, and mint leaves on the wraps.

4. Season with salt and pepper, then roll into wraps.

Nutrition Information:

- Calories: 280
- Protein: 10g
- Carbohydrates: 40g
- Fat: 10g
- Fiber: 12g
- Sugar: 5g
- Portion Size: 1 wrap

Zucchini Noodles with Pesto

Ingredients:

- 4 medium zucchinis, spiralized
- 1 cup cherry tomatoes, halved
- 1/2 cup pine nuts, toasted
- 1/2 cup fresh basil leaves
- 1/2 cup Parmesan cheese, grated
- 2 cloves garlic
- 1/2 cup olive oil
- Salt and pepper to taste

Instructions:

1. Spiralize zucchinis and set aside.

2. In a food processor, combine basil, pine nuts, Parmesan, and garlic. Pulse until finely chopped.

3. With the processor running, slowly add olive oil until the pesto is smooth.

4. Toss zucchini noodles with pesto and cherry tomatoes.

5. Season with salt and pepper before serving.

Nutrition Information:

- Calories: 280
- Protein: 8g
- Carbohydrates: 10g
- Fat: 24g
- Fiber: 4g
- Sugar: 4g
- Portion Size: 1 cup

Brown Rice and Vegetable Stir-Fry

Ingredients:

- 2 cups brown rice, cooked
- 1 cup broccoli florets
- 1 bell pepper, sliced

- 1 carrot, julienned
- 1 cup snap peas
- 1/4 cup soy sauce
- 2 tablespoons sesame oil
- 1 tablespoon ginger, minced
- 2 cloves garlic, minced

Instructions:

1. In a wok or large pan, heat sesame oil.
2. Stir-fry broccoli, bell pepper, carrot, snap peas, ginger, and garlic until crisp-tender.
3. Add cooked brown rice and soy sauce, tossing to combine.
4. Cook for an additional 3-5 minutes.

Nutrition Information:

- Calories: 320
- Protein: 10g
- Carbohydrates: 50g
- Fat: 8g
- Fiber: 8g
- Sugar: 5g

- Portion Size: 1 cup

Caprese Salad with Avocado

Ingredients:

- 4 large tomatoes, sliced
- 1 ball fresh mozzarella, sliced
- 1 avocado, sliced
- Fresh basil leaves
- Balsamic glaze
- Salt and pepper to taste

Instructions:

1. Arrange tomato and mozzarella slices on a plate.
2. Top with avocado slices and fresh basil leaves.
3. Drizzle with balsamic glaze.
4. Season with salt and pepper.

Nutrition Information:

- Calories: 200
- Protein: 10g
- Carbohydrates: 10g
- Fat: 15g

- Fiber: 5g

- Sugar: 3g

- Portion Size: 1 serving

Sweet Potato and Chickpea Curry

Ingredients:

- 2 sweet potatoes, peeled and diced

- 1 can chickpeas, drained and rinsed

- 1 onion, finely chopped

- 2 cloves garlic, minced

- 1 can coconut milk

- 2 tablespoons curry powder

- 1 teaspoon turmeric

- Salt and pepper to taste

Instructions:

1. In a pot, sauté onion and garlic until softened.

2. Add sweet potatoes, chickpeas, curry powder, turmeric, salt, and pepper.

3. Pour in coconut milk and simmer until sweet potatoes are tender.

4. Adjust seasoning before serving.

Nutrition Information:

- Calories: 300
- Protein: 10g
- Carbohydrates: 40g
- Fat: 12g
- Fiber: 8g
- Sugar: 5g
- Portion Size: 1 cup

Spinach and Quinoa Stuffed Tomatoes

Ingredients:

- 4 large tomatoes, hollowed
- 1 cup cooked quinoa
- 1 cup spinach, chopped
- 1/4 cup feta cheese, crumbled
- 1/4 cup pine nuts, toasted
- 1 tablespoon olive oil
- Salt and pepper to taste

Instructions:

1. Preheat the oven to 350°F (175°C).
2. In a bowl, combine cooked quinoa, chopped spinach, feta, pine nuts, olive oil, salt, and pepper.
3. Stuff tomatoes with the quinoa mixture.
4. Bake for 20-25 minutes.

Nutrition Information:

- Calories: 250
- Protein: 8g
- Carbohydrates: 30g
- Fat: 12g
- Fiber: 6g
- Sugar: 5g
- Portion Size: 1 stuffed tomato

Cucumber and Avocado Sushi Rolls

Ingredients:

- 2 cups sushi rice, cooked
- 4 sheets nori seaweed
- 1 cucumber, julienned
- 1 avocado, sliced

- Soy sauce for dipping

- Pickled ginger and wasabi (optional)

Instructions:

1. Place a sheet of nori on a bamboo sushi mat.

2. Spread a thin layer of sushi rice over the nori.

3. Arrange cucumber and avocado along one edge.

4. Roll tightly and slice into bite-sized pieces.

5. Serve with soy sauce and optional pickled ginger and wasabi.

Nutrition Information:

- Calories: 220

- Protein: 5g

- Carbohydrates: 40g

- Fat: 5g

- Fiber: 6g

- Sugar: 2g

- Portion Size: 6 pieces

Mediterranean Chickpea Salad

Ingredients:

- 2 cans chickpeas, drained and rinsed
- 1 cucumber, diced
- 1 cup cherry tomatoes, halved
- 1/2 red onion, finely chopped
- 1/2 cup Kalamata olives, sliced
- 1/2 cup feta cheese, crumbled
- 2 tablespoons olive oil
- 1 teaspoon dried oregano
- Salt and pepper to taste

Instructions:

1. In a large bowl, combine chickpeas, cucumber, cherry tomatoes, red onion, olives, and feta.
2. Drizzle with olive oil and sprinkle with oregano, salt, and pepper.
3. Toss gently before serving.

Nutrition Information:

- Calories: 280
- Protein: 12g

- Carbohydrates: 30g

- Fat: 14g

- Fiber: 8g

- Sugar: 5g

- Portion Size: 1 cup

Butternut Squash and Kale Salad

Ingredients:

- 1 small butternut squash, cubed

- 4 cups kale, chopped

- 1/2 cup pecans, toasted

- 1/4 cup dried cranberries

- 2 tablespoons balsamic vinegar

- 1 tablespoon olive oil

- Salt and pepper to taste

Instructions:

1. Roast butternut squash cubes until tender.

2. In a large bowl, massage kale with balsamic vinegar and olive oil.

3. Add roasted butternut squash, toasted pecans, and dried cranberries.

4. Toss well and season with salt and pepper.

Nutrition Information:

- Calories: 260
- Protein: 8g
- Carbohydrates: 40g
- Fat: 10g
- Fiber: 6g
- Sugar: 10g
- Portion Size: 1 serving

Black Bean and Corn Quesadilla

Ingredients:

- 4 whole-grain tortillas
- 1 can black beans, drained and rinsed
- 1 cup corn kernels
- 1 cup shredded cheddar cheese
- 1/2 cup salsa
- 1/4 cup cilantro, chopped
- Cooking spray

Instructions:

1. In a bowl, mix black beans, corn, cheddar cheese, salsa, and cilantro.

2. Place a tortilla on a heated skillet, add the bean mixture, and top with another tortilla.

3. Cook until the cheese melts, flipping halfway.

4. Repeat for the remaining quesadillas.

Nutrition Information:

- Calories: 320
- Protein: 15g
- Carbohydrates: 40g
- Fat: 12g
- Fiber: 8g
- Sugar: 5g
- Portion Size: 1 quesadilla

Mushroom and Lentil Lettuce Wraps

Ingredients:

- 1 cup brown lentils, cooked
- 1 cup mushrooms, chopped
- 1 bell pepper, diced

- 2 cloves garlic, minced

- 2 tablespoons soy sauce

- 1 tablespoon hoisin sauce

- 1 teaspoon sesame oil

- Lettuce leaves for wrapping

Instructions:

1. In a pan, sauté mushrooms, bell pepper, and garlic until softened.

2. Add cooked lentils, soy sauce, hoisin sauce, and sesame oil. Cook for 5 minutes.

3. Spoon the mixture into lettuce leaves to create wraps.

Nutrition Information:

- Calories: 240

- Protein: 12g

- Carbohydrates: 30g

- Fat: 6g

- Fiber: 8g

- Sugar: 4g

- Portion Size: 2 wraps

Greek Salad with Tofu Feta

Ingredients:

- 4 cups mixed salad greens
- 1 cucumber, sliced
- 1 cup cherry tomatoes, halved
- 1/2 red onion, thinly sliced
- 1/2 cup Kalamata olives
- 1/2 cup tofu feta (firm tofu, olive oil, lemon juice, dried oregano)
- Greek dressing

Instructions:

1. In a large bowl, combine salad greens, cucumber, cherry tomatoes, red onion, and olives.
2. Toss with Greek dressing.
3. Top with tofu feta.

Nutrition Information:

- Calories: 280
- Protein: 10g
- Carbohydrates: 20g
- Fat: 18g

- Fiber: 6g
- Sugar: 5g
- Portion Size: 1 serving

Chapter 4: Dinner Recipes

Dinner is a crucial part of your day, and we've crafted delicious and nutritious recipes to make your evenings both satisfying and diabetes-friendly. These recipes are thoughtfully designed to not only cater to your taste buds but also align with a vegetarian diet tailored for managing Type 2 Diabetes.

Cauliflower and Broccoli Bake

Ingredients:

- 1 medium cauliflower, chopped
- 2 cups broccoli florets
- 1 cup low-fat shredded cheddar cheese
- 1 cup unsweetened almond milk
- 2 tablespoons whole wheat flour
- 1 teaspoon Dijon mustard
- Salt and pepper to taste

Instructions:

1. Preheat the oven to 375°F (190°C).

2. Steam cauliflower and broccoli until tender.

3. In a saucepan, whisk almond milk, flour, mustard, salt, and pepper over medium heat until thickened.

4. Layer cauliflower and broccoli in a baking dish, pour the sauce over, and top with cheddar cheese.

5. Bake for 20-25 minutes or until bubbly and golden.

6. Enjoy!

Nutrition Information (per serving):

- Calories: 180
- Protein: 10g
- Carbohydrates: 15g
- Fat: 8g
- Fiber: 5g
- Sugar: 3g
- Portion Size: 1 cup

Portobello Mushroom Steaks

Ingredients:

- 4 large portobello mushrooms, cleaned
- 2 tablespoons balsamic vinegar
- 2 tablespoons olive oil

- 2 cloves garlic, minced

- 1 teaspoon dried thyme

- Salt and pepper to taste

Instructions:

1. Preheat the grill or grill pan.

2. Mix balsamic vinegar, olive oil, garlic, thyme, salt, and pepper to create a marinade.

3. Brush the mushroom caps with the marinade and grill for 5-7 minutes per side.

4. Serve hot.

Nutrition Information (per serving):

- Calories: 120

- Protein: 4g

- Carbohydrates: 8g

- Fat: 10g

- Fiber: 2g

- Sugar: 4g

- Portion Size: 1 mushroom

Ratatouille with Quinoa

Ingredients:

- 1 eggplant, diced
- 1 zucchini, sliced
- 1 yellow bell pepper, diced
- 1 red onion, chopped
- 2 cloves garlic, minced
- 1 can (14 oz) diced tomatoes
- 1 teaspoon dried thyme
- 1 teaspoon dried rosemary
- Salt and pepper to taste
- 1 cup cooked quinoa

Instructions:

1. Preheat the oven to 375°F (190°C).
2. In a baking dish, layer eggplant, zucchini, bell pepper, onion, and garlic.
3. Pour diced tomatoes over the vegetables, sprinkle with thyme, rosemary, salt, and pepper.
4. Bake for 30-35 minutes until vegetables are tender.
5. Serve over a bed of cooked quinoa.

Nutrition Information (per serving):

- Calories: 220
- Protein: 6g
- Carbohydrates: 40g
- Fat: 4g
- Fiber: 8g
- Sugar: 10g
- Portion Size: 1 cup

Spaghetti Squash Primavera

Ingredients:

- 1 medium spaghetti squash, halved
- 2 tablespoons olive oil
- 2 cloves garlic, minced
- 1 cup cherry tomatoes, halved
- 1 cup baby spinach
- 1/4 cup grated Parmesan cheese
- Salt and pepper to taste

Instructions:

1. Preheat the oven to 375°F (190°C).
2. Scoop out the seeds from the spaghetti squash halves.

3. Brush with olive oil, sprinkle with salt and pepper, and roast for 40-45 minutes.

4. In a pan, sauté garlic, add tomatoes and spinach until wilted.

5. Scrape the spaghetti squash with a fork to create "noodles," mix with the sautéed vegetables.

6. Top with Parmesan cheese and serve.

Nutrition Information (per serving):

- Calories: 180
- Protein: 5g
- Carbohydrates: 22g
- Fat: 9g
- Fiber: 6g
- Sugar: 8g
- Portion Size: 1 cup

Thai Red Curry with Tofu

Ingredients:

- 1 block extra-firm tofu, cubed
- 1 tablespoon red curry paste
- 1 can (14 oz) coconut milk

- 1 cup broccoli florets
- 1 red bell pepper, sliced
- 1 carrot, julienned
- 2 tablespoons soy sauce
- 1 tablespoon coconut sugar
- Fresh cilantro for garnish

Instructions:

1. In a pan, sauté tofu until golden brown.
2. Add red curry paste, coconut milk, broccoli, bell pepper, carrot, soy sauce, and coconut sugar.
3. Simmer for 15-20 minutes until vegetables are tender.
4. Garnish with fresh cilantro and serve over brown rice or quinoa.

Nutrition Information (per serving):
- Calories: 280
- Protein: 14g
- Carbohydrates: 18g
- Fat: 18g
- Fiber: 5g

- Sugar: 8g
- Portion Size: 1 cup

Eggplant Parmesan

Ingredients:

- 2 medium eggplants, sliced
- 1 cup whole wheat breadcrumbs
- 1 cup marinara sauce (low sugar)
- 1 cup part-skim mozzarella cheese, shredded
- 1/4 cup grated Parmesan cheese
- Fresh basil for garnish

Instructions:

1. Preheat the oven to 375°F (190°C).
2. Coat eggplant slices with breadcrumbs and bake until golden brown.
3. In a baking dish, layer baked eggplant, marinara sauce, mozzarella, and Parmesan.
4. Repeat layers and bake for 25-30 minutes.
5. Garnish with fresh basil and serve.

Nutrition Information (per serving):

- Calories: 220
- Protein: 12g
- Carbohydrates: 25g
- Fat: 9g
- Fiber: 9g
- Sugar: 8g
- Portion Size: 1 cup

Stuffed Acorn Squash with Wild Rice

Ingredients:

- 4 acorn squash, halved
- 1 cup wild rice, cooked
- 1 cup black beans, drained and rinsed
- 1 cup corn kernels
- 1/2 cup red onion, diced
- 1 teaspoon cumin
- 1 teaspoon chili powder
- Salt and pepper to taste

Instructions:

1. Preheat the oven to 400°F (200°C).

2. Place acorn squash halves on a baking sheet, roast for 30-35 minutes.

3. In a bowl, mix cooked wild rice, black beans, corn, red onion, cumin, chili powder, salt, and pepper.

4. Stuff each acorn squash half with the mixture.

5. Bake for an additional 15 minutes and serve.

Nutrition Information (per serving):

- Calories: 280
- Protein: 10g
- Carbohydrates: 58g
- Fat: 2g
- Fiber: 10g
- Sugar: 3g
- Portion Size: 1 half squash

Cabbage and Lentil Casserole

Ingredients:

- 1 cup green lentils, cooked
- 1 small head cabbage, shredded
- 1 onion, chopped
- 2 cloves garlic, minced

- 1 can (14 oz) diced tomatoes

- 1 teaspoon smoked paprika

- 1 teaspoon dried thyme

- Salt and pepper to taste

Instructions:

1. Preheat the oven to 375°F (190°C).

2. In a skillet, sauté onion and garlic until translucent.

3. Add lentils, cabbage, diced tomatoes, smoked paprika, thyme, salt, and pepper.

4. Transfer to a baking dish and bake for 30-35 minutes.

5. Enjoy!

Nutrition Information (per serving):

- Calories: 240

- Protein: 14g

- Carbohydrates: 45g

- Fat: 1g

- Fiber: 15g

- Sugar: 8g

- Portion Size: 1 cup

Quinoa-stuffed Bell Peppers

Ingredients:

- 4 bell peppers, halved
- 1 cup quinoa, cooked
- 1 can (14 oz) black beans, drained and rinsed
- 1 cup corn kernels
- 1 cup salsa (no added sugar)
- 1 teaspoon ground cumin
- 1 teaspoon chili powder
- Salt and pepper to taste

Instructions:

1. Preheat the oven to 375°F (190°C).
2. Boil bell pepper halves for 5 minutes.
3. In a bowl, mix quinoa, black beans, corn, salsa, cumin, chili powder, salt, and pepper.
4. Stuff each bell pepper half with the quinoa mixture.
5. Bake for 20-25 minutes and serve.

Nutrition Information (per serving):

- Calories: 290
- Protein: 13g

- Carbohydrates: 55g

- Fat: 2g

- Fiber: 12g

- Sugar: 8g

- Portion Size: 1 half pepper

Sweet Potato and Black Bean Enchiladas

Ingredients:

- 2 large sweet potatoes, diced

- 1 can (14 oz) black beans, mashed

- 1 cup corn kernels

- 1 red onion, diced

- 8 whole wheat tortillas

- 1 cup enchilada sauce (no added sugar)

- 1 cup shredded cheddar cheese

- Fresh cilantro for garnish

Instructions:

1. Preheat the oven to 375°F (190°C).

2. Roast sweet potatoes until tender.

3. In a bowl, mix mashed black beans, corn, roasted sweet potatoes, and diced red onion.

4. Spoon the mixture onto each tortilla, roll, and place in a baking dish.

5. Pour enchilada sauce over the rolled tortillas, sprinkle with cheddar cheese.

6. Bake for 20-25 minutes, garnish with fresh cilantro, and serve.

Nutrition Information (per serving):

- Calories: 320
- Protein: 15g
- Carbohydrates: 50g
- Fat: 8g
- Fiber: 12g
- Sugar: 8g
- Portion Size: 2 enchiladas

Mushroom and Spinach Lasagna

Ingredients:

- 9 whole wheat lasagna noodles, cooked
- 2 cups mushrooms, sliced

- 4 cups baby spinach

- 2 cups ricotta cheese (part-skim)

- 1 cup marinara sauce (low sugar)

- 1 cup mozzarella cheese, shredded

- 1/4 cup grated Parmesan cheese

- Fresh basil for garnish

Instructions:

1. Preheat the oven to 375°F (190°C).

2. In a pan, sauté mushrooms until golden, add spinach until wilted.

3. In a baking dish, layer noodles, ricotta, mushroom-spinach mixture, marinara, and cheeses.

4. Repeat layers and bake for 30-35 minutes.

5. Garnish with fresh basil and serve.

Nutrition Information (per serving):

- Calories: 330

- Protein: 20g

- Carbohydrates: 35g

- Fat: 12g

- Fiber: 5g

- Sugar: 6g
- Portion Size: 1 square

Teriyaki Tofu Stir-Fry

Ingredients:

- 1 block extra-firm tofu, cubed
- 2 cups broccoli florets
- 1 red bell pepper, sliced
- 1 carrot, julienned
- 1 cup snow peas
- 1/2 cup low-sodium teriyaki sauce
- 2 tablespoons sesame oil
- 2 cloves garlic, minced
- 1 teaspoon ginger, grated
- Sesame seeds for garnish

Instructions:

1. In a wok or large skillet, sauté tofu until golden brown.
2. Add broccoli, bell pepper, carrot, and snow peas. Stir-fry for 5-7 minutes.

3. In a bowl, mix teriyaki sauce, sesame oil, garlic, and ginger. Pour over the tofu-vegetable mixture.

4. Continue stir-frying until the sauce thickens.

5. Garnish with sesame seeds and serve over brown rice.

Nutrition Information (per serving):

- Calories: 280
- Protein: 15g
- Carbohydrates: 30g
- Fat: 12g
- Fiber: 8g
- Sugar: 10g
- Portion Size: 1 cup

Lentil and Vegetable Curry

Ingredients:

- 1 cup dry green lentils, cooked
- 1 cup cauliflower florets
- 1 cup carrots, sliced
- 1 cup green beans, cut into pieces
- 1 onion, chopped

- 2 cloves garlic, minced
- 1 can (14 oz) coconut milk
- 2 tablespoons curry powder
- Salt and pepper to taste

Instructions:

1. In a pot, sauté onion and garlic until translucent.
2. Add cooked lentils, cauliflower, carrots, green beans, coconut milk, curry powder, salt, and pepper.
3. Simmer for 20-25 minutes until vegetables are tender.
4. Serve over brown rice or quinoa.

Nutrition Information (per serving):

- Calories: 310
- Protein: 15g
- Carbohydrates: 45g
- Fat: 8g
- Fiber: 14g
- Sugar: 5g
- Portion Size: 1 cup

Spinach and Ricotta Stuffed Shells

Ingredients:

- 18 jumbo pasta shells, cooked
- 2 cups baby spinach, chopped
- 2 cups ricotta cheese (part-skim)
- 1 egg
- 1/2 cup grated Parmesan cheese
- 2 cups marinara sauce (low sugar)
- 1 cup mozzarella cheese, shredded
- Fresh basil for garnish

Instructions:

1. Preheat the oven to 375°F (190°C).
2. In a bowl, mix chopped spinach, ricotta, egg, and Parmesan.
3. Stuff each pasta shell with the spinach-ricotta mixture.
4. In a baking dish, spread marinara sauce, arrange stuffed shells, and sprinkle with mozzarella.
5. Bake for 25-30 minutes.
6. Garnish with fresh basil and serve.

Nutrition Information (per serving):

- Calories: 340
- Protein: 18g
- Carbohydrates: 35g
- Fat: 15g
- Fiber: 5g
- Sugar: 7g
- Portion Size: 3 shells

Vegan Chili with Kidney Beans

Ingredients:

- 2 cans (15 oz each) kidney beans, drained and rinsed
- 1 can (14 oz) diced tomatoes
- 1 cup corn kernels
- 1 onion, diced
- 2 cloves garlic, minced
- 1 bell pepper, diced
- 1 zucchini, diced
- 2 tablespoons chili powder
- 1 teaspoon cumin
- Salt and pepper to taste

Instructions:

1. In a pot, sauté onion and garlic until translucent.

2. Add kidney beans, diced tomatoes, corn, bell pepper, zucchini, chili powder, cumin, salt, and pepper.

3. Simmer for 30-35 minutes.

4. Serve hot.

Nutrition Information (per serving):

- Calories: 270
- Protein: 15g
- Carbohydrates: 50g
- Fat: 1g
- Fiber: 14g
- Sugar: 7g
- Portion Size: 1 cup

Chapter 5: Snacks and Appetizers

These delectable recipes are designed to offer a delightful balance of flavors and nutrition. Whether you're hosting a gathering or simply treating yourself, these snacks and appetizers are sure to satisfy. Dive into the culinary journey that awaits you!

Guacamole with Veggie Sticks

Ingredients:

- 3 ripe avocados
- 1 small onion, finely diced
- 1-2 tomatoes, diced
- 1 clove garlic, minced
- Fresh cilantro, chopped
- Lime juice, to taste
- Salt and pepper, to taste

Instructions:

1. Mash avocados in a bowl.
2. Add diced onion, tomatoes, garlic, and cilantro.

3. Squeeze lime juice over the mixture.

4. Season with salt and pepper.

5. Serve with an assortment of fresh veggie sticks.

Nutrition Information (per serving):

- Calories: 120

- Protein: 2g

- Carbohydrates: 7g

- Fat: 10g

- Fiber: 5g

- Sugar: 1g

- Portion size: 1/2 cup guacamole with veggie sticks.

Edamame Hummus with Whole Grain Crackers

Ingredients:

- 1 cup shelled edamame, cooked

- 1 can chickpeas, drained

- 2 cloves garlic

- 3 tablespoons tahini

- 2 tablespoons olive oil

- Lemon juice, to taste
- Salt and cumin, to taste

Instructions:

1. Blend edamame, chickpeas, garlic, tahini, and olive oil in a food processor.
2. Add lemon juice, salt, and cumin to taste.
3. Blend until smooth.
4. Serve with whole grain crackers.

Nutrition Information (per serving):

- Calories: 150
- Protein: 6g
- Carbohydrates: 12g
- Fat: 9g
- Fiber: 4g
- Sugar: 1g
- Portion size: 1/4 cup hummus with whole grain crackers.

Roasted Chickpeas with Cumin

Ingredients:

- 2 cans chickpeas, drained and rinsed
- 2 tablespoons olive oil
- 1 teaspoon cumin
- Salt and pepper, to taste

Instructions:

1. Preheat oven to 400°F (200°C).
2. Toss chickpeas with olive oil, cumin, salt, and pepper.
3. Spread on a baking sheet.
4. Roast for 25-30 minutes, until crispy.
5. Allow to cool before serving.

Nutrition Information (per serving):

- Calories: 120
- Protein: 5g
- Carbohydrates: 18g
- Fat: 3g
- Fiber: 5g
- Sugar: 1g

- Portion size: 1/2 cup roasted chickpeas.

Greek Yogurt and Berry Parfait

Ingredients:

- 1 cup Greek yogurt
- Mixed berries (strawberries, blueberries, raspberries)
- Honey, to taste
- Granola

Instructions:

1. Layer Greek yogurt in a glass or bowl.
2. Add mixed berries on top.
3. Drizzle with honey.
4. Sprinkle granola over the top.

Nutrition Information (per serving):

- Calories: 180
- Protein: 15g
- Carbohydrates: 25g
- Fat: 4g
- Fiber: 3g
- Sugar: 15g

- Portion size: 1 cup parfait.

Sliced Apple with Almond Butter

Ingredients:

- 1 apple, sliced
- 2 tablespoons almond butter

Instructions:

1. Arrange apple slices on a plate.
2. Serve with almond butter for dipping.

Nutrition Information (per serving):

- Calories: 180
- Protein: 3g
- Carbohydrates: 20g
- Fat: 10g
- Fiber: 5g
- Sugar: 12g
- Portion size: 1 sliced apple with almond butter.

Veggie Spring Rolls with Peanut Sauce

Ingredients:

- Rice paper wrappers
- Mixed vegetables (carrots, bell peppers, cucumber)
- Fresh herbs (mint, cilantro)
- Rice noodles, cooked
- Peanut sauce for dipping

Instructions:

1. Soak rice paper wrappers in warm water until pliable.
2. Fill with a combination of vegetables and herbs.
3. Add a small portion of cooked rice noodles.
4. Roll tightly and serve with peanut sauce.

Nutrition Information (per serving):

- Calories: 120
- Protein: 3g
- Carbohydrates: 25g
- Fat: 1g
- Fiber: 3g
- Sugar: 2g

- Portion size: 2 spring rolls with peanut sauce.

Caprese Skewers with Balsamic Glaze

Ingredients:

- Cherry tomatoes
- Fresh mozzarella balls
- Fresh basil leaves
- Balsamic glaze

Instructions:

1. Thread a cherry tomato, mozzarella ball, and basil leaf onto skewers.
2. Arrange on a serving platter.
3. Drizzle with balsamic glaze before serving.

Nutrition Information (per serving):

- Calories: 90
- Protein: 5g
- Carbohydrates: 3g
- Fat: 6g

- Fiber: 1g

- Sugar: 2g

- Portion size: 3 skewers.

Almond and Coconut Energy Bites

Ingredients:

- 1 cup almonds, finely ground

- 1/2 cup shredded coconut

- 1/4 cup almond butter

- 2 tablespoons honey

- 1 teaspoon vanilla extract

- Pinch of salt

Instructions:

1. Combine ground almonds, shredded coconut, almond butter, honey, vanilla extract, and salt in a bowl.

2. Mix until well combined.

3. Roll into bite-sized balls.

4. Chill in the refrigerator before serving.

Nutrition Information (per serving):

- Calories: 80
- Protein: 3g
- Carbohydrates: 6g
- Fat: 6g
- Fiber: 2g
- Sugar: 3g
- Portion size: 2 energy bites.

Stuffed Mini Bell Peppers with Herbed Cream Cheese

Ingredients:

- Mini bell peppers
- Cream cheese, softened
- Fresh herbs (parsley, chives, dill)
- Garlic powder
- Salt and pepper, to taste

Instructions:

1. Cut mini bell peppers in half, removing seeds.

2. In a bowl, mix cream cheese with chopped herbs, garlic powder, salt, and pepper.

3. Stuff each pepper half with the herbed cream cheese mixture.

Nutrition Information (per serving):

- Calories: 70

- Protein: 2g

- Carbohydrates: 5g

- Fat: 5g

- Fiber: 1g

- Sugar: 3g

- Portion size: 4 stuffed pepper halves.

Sweet Potato Fries with Avocado Dip

Ingredients:

- Sweet potatoes, cut into fries

- Olive oil

- Paprika

- Salt and pepper, to taste

- Avocado, mashed

Instructions:

1. Toss sweet potato fries with olive oil, paprika, salt, and pepper.
2. Bake until crispy.
3. Serve with mashed avocado for dipping.

Nutrition Information (per serving):

- Calories: 160
- Protein: 2g
- Carbohydrates: 20g
- Fat: 9g
- Fiber: 5g
- Sugar: 3g
- Portion size: 1 cup sweet potato fries with avocado dip.

Cucumber Cups with Tzatziki

Ingredients:

- English cucumbers
- Greek yogurt

- Garlic, minced

- Fresh dill, chopped

- Lemon juice

- Salt and pepper, to taste

Instructions:

1. Cut cucumbers into thick slices.

2. Scoop out the center to create cups.

3. Mix Greek yogurt with garlic, dill, lemon juice, salt, and pepper.

4. Fill cucumber cups with tzatziki.

Nutrition Information (per serving):

- Calories: 50

- Protein: 3g

- Carbohydrates: 7g

- Fat: 2g

- Fiber: 1g

- Sugar: 4g

- Portion size: 4 cucumber cups with tzatziki.

Avocado and Black Bean Salsa

Ingredients:

- 2 ripe avocados, diced

- 1 can black beans, drained and rinsed

- Corn kernels (fresh or canned), cooked

- Red onion, finely chopped

- Fresh cilantro, chopped

- Lime juice

- Salt and pepper, to taste

Instructions:

1. In a bowl, combine diced avocados, black beans, corn, red onion, and cilantro.

2. Squeeze lime juice over the mixture.

3. Season with salt and pepper.

4. Gently toss and refrigerate before serving.

Nutrition Information (per serving):

- Calories: 130

- Protein: 5g

- Carbohydrates: 17g

- Fat: 6g

- Fiber: 7g

- Sugar: 1g

- Portion size: 1/2 cup avocado and black bean salsa.

Tomato Basil Bruschetta

Ingredients:

- Tomatoes, diced

- Fresh basil, chopped

- Garlic, minced

- Olive oil

- Balsamic vinegar

- Salt and pepper, to taste

- Whole grain baguette slices

Instructions:

1. In a bowl, combine diced tomatoes, basil, garlic, olive oil, and balsamic vinegar.

2. Season with salt and pepper.

3. Toast whole grain baguette slices and top with the tomato mixture.

Nutrition Information (per serving):

- Calories: 90
- Protein: 2g
- Carbohydrates: 15g
- Fat: 3g
- Fiber: 2g
- Sugar: 2g
- Portion size: 2 slices of bruschetta.

Mixed Nuts and Seeds Trail Mix

Ingredients:

- Almonds
- Walnuts
- Pumpkin seeds
- Sunflower seeds
- Dried cranberries
- Dark chocolate chips

Instructions:

1. Mix almonds, walnuts, pumpkin seeds, sunflower seeds, dried cranberries, and dark chocolate chips in a bowl.

2. Adjust quantities to your liking.

3. Store in an airtight container for a convenient snack.

Nutrition Information (per serving):

- Calories: 180

- Protein: 6g

- Carbohydrates: 14g

- Fat: 12g

- Fiber: 3g

- Sugar: 7g

- Portion size: 1/4 cup trail mix.

Roasted Red Pepper Hummus with Pita Chips

Ingredients:

- 1 can chickpeas, drained

- Roasted red peppers

- Garlic, minced

- Tahini

- Lemon juice

- Olive oil

- Paprika

- Salt and pepper, to taste

- Whole grain pita, cut into triangles

Instructions:

1. Blend chickpeas, roasted red peppers, garlic, tahini, lemon juice, olive oil, paprika, salt, and pepper in a food processor until smooth.

2. Serve with whole grain pita chips.

Nutrition Information (per serving):

- Calories: 160

- Protein: 5g

- Carbohydrates: 22g

- Fat: 7g

- Fiber: 5g

- Sugar: 2g

- Portion size: 1/4 cup hummus with pita chips.

Chapter 6: Desserts

These dessert recipes not only satisfy your sweet tooth but also adhere to the principles of a healthy lifestyle. Packed with wholesome ingredients and mindful preparation, these desserts promise a delightful culinary journey without compromising on taste or nutrition.

Berry and Chia Seed Popsicles

Ingredients:

- 1 cup mixed berries (strawberries, blueberries, raspberries)
- 2 tablespoons chia seeds
- 1 tablespoon honey
- 1 cup unsweetened almond milk

Instructions:

1. Blend berries, chia seeds, and almond milk until smooth.
2. Stir in honey and pour the mixture into popsicle molds.

3. Freeze for at least 4 hours.

4. Enjoy these refreshing popsicles guilt-free!

Nutrition Information (per serving):

- Calories: 80

- Protein: 2g

- Carbohydrates: 15g

- Fat: 2g

- Fiber: 5g

- Sugar: 8g

- Portion Size: 1 popsicle

Dark Chocolate-Dipped Strawberries

Ingredients:

- 1 cup dark chocolate chips

- 1 pint fresh strawberries, washed and dried

Instructions:

1. Melt dark chocolate in a heatproof bowl.

2. Dip each strawberry into the melted chocolate.

3. Place on parchment paper and refrigerate until the chocolate hardens.

4. A guilt-free indulgence!

Nutrition Information (per serving):

- Calories: 60

- Protein: 1g

- Carbohydrates: 10g

- Fat: 4g

- Fiber: 2g

- Sugar: 6g

- Portion Size: 3 strawberries

Baked Apple with Cinnamon

Ingredients:

- 2 medium-sized apples, cored and sliced

- 1 teaspoon cinnamon

- 1 tablespoon honey

Instructions:

1. Preheat the oven to 375°F (190°C).

2. Place apple slices in a baking dish.

3. Sprinkle with cinnamon and drizzle honey.

4. Bake for 20-25 minutes until apples are tender.

5. A warm and comforting treat!

Nutrition Information (per serving):

- Calories: 90
- Protein: 1g
- Carbohydrates: 24g
- Fat: 0g
- Fiber: 5g
- Sugar: 18g
- Portion Size: 1 apple

Avocado Chocolate Mousse

Ingredients:

- 2 ripe avocados
- 1/4 cup unsweetened cocoa powder
- 1/4 cup honey
- 1 teaspoon vanilla extract

Instructions:

1. Blend avocados, cocoa powder, honey, and vanilla until smooth.
2. Refrigerate for at least 2 hours before serving.

3. A rich and creamy chocolate delight!

Nutrition Information (per serving):

- Calories: 150
- Protein: 2g
- Carbohydrates: 18g
- Fat: 10g
- Fiber: 7g
- Sugar: 9g
- Portion Size: 1/2 cup

Coconut and Berry Sorbet

Ingredients:

- 2 cups mixed berries
- 1 can (14 oz) coconut milk
- 1/4 cup maple syrup

Instructions:

1. Blend berries, coconut milk, and maple syrup until smooth.
2. Pour into a shallow dish and freeze for 4 hours.
3. Scoop out and enjoy this refreshing sorbet!

Nutrition Information (per serving):

- Calories: 120
- Protein: 1g
- Carbohydrates: 18g
- Fat: 6g
- Fiber: 4g
- Sugar: 12g
- Portion Size: 1/2 cup

Pumpkin Pie Smoothie

Ingredients:

- 1/2 cup canned pumpkin puree
- 1 banana
- 1/2 teaspoon pumpkin pie spice
- 1 cup unsweetened almond milk
- Ice cubes

Instructions:

1. Blend pumpkin puree, banana, pumpkin pie spice, and almond milk until smooth.
2. Add ice cubes and blend again.
3. A seasonal, guilt-free smoothie treat!

Nutrition Information (per serving):

- Calories: 100
- Protein: 2g
- Carbohydrates: 20g
- Fat: 2g
- Fiber: 5g
- Sugar: 9g
- Portion Size: 1 cup

Almond Flour Blueberry Muffins

Ingredients:

- 2 cups almond flour
- 1/2 teaspoon baking soda
- 1/4 teaspoon salt
- 3 eggs
- 1/4 cup coconut oil, melted
- 1/4 cup honey
- 1 teaspoon vanilla extract
- 1 cup fresh blueberries

Instructions:

1. Preheat the oven to 350°F (175°C) and line a muffin tin.

2. In a bowl, mix almond flour, baking soda, and salt.

3. In another bowl, whisk eggs, coconut oil, honey, and vanilla.

4. Combine wet and dry ingredients, then fold in blueberries.

5. Spoon batter into muffin cups and bake for 20-25 minutes.

6. Enjoy these moist and flavorful muffins!

Nutrition Information (per serving):

- Calories: 180
- Protein: 5g
- Carbohydrates: 14g
- Fat: 12g
- Fiber: 3g
- Sugar: 8g
- Portion Size: 1 muffin

Banana and Walnut Bread

Ingredients:

- 2 ripe bananas, mashed
- 1/4 cup coconut oil, melted
- 1/4 cup honey
- 2 eggs
- 1 teaspoon vanilla extract
- 1 3/4 cups whole wheat flour
- 1/2 teaspoon baking soda
- 1/4 teaspoon salt
- 1/2 cup chopped walnuts

Instructions:

1. Preheat the oven to 350°F (175°C) and grease a loaf pan.
2. In a bowl, mix mashed bananas, coconut oil, honey, eggs, and vanilla.
3. In another bowl, combine flour, baking soda, and salt.
4. Gradually add dry ingredients to wet, then fold in walnuts.

5. Pour batter into the loaf pan and bake for 55-60 minutes.

6. A wholesome and nutty banana bread!

Nutrition Information (per serving):

- Calories: 180

- Protein: 4g

- Carbohydrates: 22g

- Fat: 9g

- Fiber: 3g

- Sugar: 10g

- Portion Size: 1 slice

Greek Yogurt and Honey Parfait

Ingredients:

- 1 cup Greek yogurt

- 2 tablespoons honey

- 1/2 cup granola

- 1/2 cup mixed berries

Instructions:

1. In a glass, layer Greek yogurt, honey, granola, and berries.
2. Repeat the layers.
3. A delightful parfait for a guilt-free indulgence!

Nutrition Information (per serving):

*   Calories: 250
*   Protein: 10g
*   Carbohydrates: 40g
*   Fat: 6g
*   Fiber: 4g
*   Sugar: 18g
*   Portion Size: 1 serving

Mango and Coconut Chia Pudding

Ingredients:

*   1/4 cup chia seeds
*   1 cup coconut milk
*   1 tablespoon honey
*   1 ripe mango, diced

Instructions:

1. Mix chia seeds, coconut milk, and honey in a bowl.

2. Refrigerate for at least 4 hours or overnight.

3. Top with diced mango before serving.

4. A tropical and nutrient-rich pudding!

Nutrition Information (per serving):

- Calories: 180

- Protein: 4g

- Carbohydrates: 22g

- Fat: 9g

- Fiber: 8g

- Sugar: 12g

- Portion Size: 1/2 cup

Raspberry Oat Bars

Ingredients:

- 2 cups rolled oats

- 1 cup whole wheat flour

- 1/2 cup coconut oil, melted

- 1/2 cup maple syrup

- 1 cup raspberry jam (no added sugar)

Instructions:

1. Preheat the oven to 350°F (175°C) and line a baking dish.
2. In a bowl, mix oats, flour, coconut oil, and maple syrup.
3. Press half of the mixture into the bottom of the dish.
4. Spread raspberry jam over the mixture.
5. Sprinkle the remaining oat mixture on top.
6. Bake for 30-35 minutes.
7. Cut into bars once cooled.

Nutrition Information (per serving):

- Calories: 160
- Protein: 3g
- Carbohydrates: 25g
- Fat: 6g
- Fiber: 3g
- Sugar: 10g
- Portion Size: 1 bar

Quinoa Chocolate Chip Cookies

Ingredients:

- 1 cup cooked quinoa, cooled
- 1 cup almond flour
- 1/2 teaspoon baking soda
- 1/4 teaspoon salt
- 1/4 cup coconut oil, melted
- 1/4 cup maple syrup
- 1 teaspoon vanilla extract
- 1/2 cup dark chocolate chips

Instructions:

1. Preheat the oven to 350°F (175°C) and line a baking sheet.
2. In a bowl, mix quinoa, almond flour, baking soda, and salt.
3. In another bowl, whisk coconut oil, maple syrup, and vanilla.
4. Combine wet and dry ingredients, then fold in chocolate chips.
5. Drop spoonfuls of dough onto the baking sheet.
6. Bake for 12-15 minutes.

7. A guilt-free twist on a classic treat!

Nutrition Information (per serving):

- Calories: 120

- Protein: 2g

- Carbohydrates: 14g

- Fat: 6g

- Fiber: 2g

- Sugar: 7g

- Portion Size: 2 cookies

Pistachio and Cranberry Energy Balls

Ingredients:

- 1 cup shelled pistachios

- 1/2 cup dried cranberries

- 1/4 cup rolled oats

- 2 tablespoons honey

- 1 teaspoon vanilla extract

Instructions:

1. In a food processor, blend pistachios, cranberries, oats, honey, and vanilla until a sticky mixture forms.
2. Roll into bite-sized balls.
3. Refrigerate for at least 30 minutes.
4. A nutrient-packed energy boost!

Nutrition Information (per serving):

- Calories: 90
- Protein: 2g
- Carbohydrates: 12g
- Fat: 4g
- Fiber: 2g
- Sugar: 7g
- Portion Size: 3 balls

Lemon Poppy Seed Cake

Ingredients:

- 1 1/2 cups almond flour
- 1/2 cup coconut flour
- 1/2 teaspoon baking soda
- 1/4 teaspoon salt

- 1/4 cup coconut oil, melted

- 1/4 cup honey

- 3 eggs

- 1/4 cup fresh lemon juice

- Zest of one lemon

- 1 tablespoon poppy seeds

Instructions:

1. Preheat the oven to 350°F (175°C) and grease a cake pan.

2. In a bowl, mix almond flour, coconut flour, baking soda, and salt.

3. In another bowl, whisk coconut oil, honey, eggs, lemon juice, lemon zest, and poppy seeds.

4. Combine wet and dry ingredients.

5. Pour batter into the cake pan and bake for 25-30 minutes.

6. A zesty and moist cake!

Nutrition Information (per serving):

- Calories: 160

- Protein: 4g

- Carbohydrates: 14g

- Fat: 10g

- Fiber: 3g

- Sugar: 7g

- Portion Size: 1 slice

Vegan Chocolate Avocado Cake

Ingredients:

- 2 ripe avocados

- 1 1/2 cups whole wheat flour

- 1/3 cup unsweetened cocoa powder

- 1 teaspoon baking soda

- 1/2 teaspoon salt

- 1 cup coconut sugar

- 1 cup water

- 1 teaspoon vanilla extract

- 1 tablespoon apple cider vinegar

Instructions:

1. Preheat the oven to 350°F (175°C) and grease a cake pan.

2. In a blender, combine avocados, flour, cocoa powder, baking soda, salt, coconut sugar, water, vanilla, and vinegar until smooth.

3. Pour batter into the cake pan and bake for 30-35 minutes.

4. A rich and decadent chocolate cake!

Nutrition Information (per serving):

- Calories: 180
- Protein: 3g
- Carbohydrates: 24g
- Fat: 9g
- Fiber: 4g
- Sugar: 12g
- Portion Size: 1 slice

Chapter 7: Smoothies

These vibrant concoctions not only tantalize the taste buds but also contribute to your well-being. Packed with a kaleidoscope of flavors, each smoothie is a testament to the art of blending wholesome ingredients into a symphony of taste and nutrition.

Green Detox Smoothie

Ingredients:

- 1 cup spinach
- 1/2 cucumber, peeled
- 1 green apple, cored
- 1/2 lemon, juiced
- 1 cup coconut water
- Ice cubes (optional)

Instructions:

1. Combine spinach, cucumber, green apple, and lemon juice in a blender.
2. Add coconut water and blend until smooth.

3. Add ice cubes if desired and blend again.

4. Pour into a glass and enjoy!

Nutrition Information:

- Calories: 120
- Protein: 3g
- Carbohydrates: 26g
- Fat: 1g
- Fiber: 6g
- Sugar: 15g
- Portion Size: 1 serving

Berry Blast Smoothie

Ingredients:

- 1 cup mixed berries (strawberries, blueberries, raspberries)
- 1/2 cup Greek yogurt
- 1/2 banana
- 1 tablespoon honey
- 1 cup almond milk
- Ice cubes (optional)

Instructions:

1. Combine mixed berries, Greek yogurt, banana, and honey in a blender.
2. Add almond milk and blend until smooth.
3. Add ice cubes if desired and blend again.
4. Pour into a glass and savor the berry goodness!

Nutrition Information:

- Calories: 180
- Protein: 7g
- Carbohydrates: 32g
- Fat: 3g
- Fiber: 5g
- Sugar: 20g
- Portion Size: 1 serving

Mango and Spinach Smoothie

Ingredients:

- 1 cup mango chunks
- 1 cup fresh spinach
- 1/2 cup plain yogurt
- 1 tablespoon chia seeds

- 1/2 lime, juiced
- 1 cup water
- Ice cubes (optional)

Instructions:

1. Blend mango chunks, fresh spinach, plain yogurt, and chia seeds.
2. Squeeze in lime juice and add water.
3. Blend until smooth and creamy.
4. Add ice cubes if desired, blend once more, and indulge!

Nutrition Information:

- Calories: 160
- Protein: 5g
- Carbohydrates: 28g
- Fat: 4g
- Fiber: 6g
- Sugar: 20g
- Portion Size: 1 serving

Pineapple and Kale Smoothie

Ingredients:

- 1 cup pineapple chunks
- 1 cup kale leaves, stems removed
- 1/2 banana
- 1/2 cup coconut milk
- 1 tablespoon flaxseeds
- Ice cubes (optional)

Instructions:

1. Combine pineapple chunks, kale leaves, banana, and coconut milk in a blender.
2. Add flaxseeds and blend until smooth.
3. Include ice cubes if desired and blend again.
4. Pour into a glass, sip, and revel in the tropical goodness!

Nutrition Information:

- Calories: 140
- Protein: 4g
- Carbohydrates: 25g
- Fat: 5g

- Fiber: 7g
- Sugar: 15g
- Portion Size: 1 serving

Banana and Almond Milk Smoothie

Ingredients:

- 2 ripe bananas
- 1 cup almond milk
- 1 tablespoon almond butter
- 1/2 teaspoon cinnamon
- 1 tablespoon hemp seeds
- Ice cubes (optional)

Instructions:

1. Blend ripe bananas, almond milk, almond butter, and cinnamon.
2. Add hemp seeds and blend until creamy.
3. Incorporate ice cubes if desired, blend once more, and enjoy the velvety texture.

Nutrition Information:

- Calories: 200

- Protein: 5g

- Carbohydrates: 30g

- Fat: 8g

- Fiber: 5g

- Sugar: 15g

- Portion Size: 1 serving

Avocado and Coconut Water Smoothie

Ingredients:

- 1 ripe avocado

- 1 cup coconut water

- 1/2 cup pineapple chunks

- 1 tablespoon lime juice

- 1 tablespoon honey

- Ice cubes (optional)

Instructions:

1. Blend ripe avocado, coconut water, pineapple chunks, lime juice, and honey.

2. Blend until smooth and creamy.

3. Add ice cubes if desired, blend once more, and experience the tropical bliss.

Nutrition Information:

- Calories: 220
- Protein: 3g
- Carbohydrates: 30g
- Fat: 12g
- Fiber: 7g
- Sugar: 18g
- Portion Size: 1 serving

Citrus Burst Smoothie

Ingredients:

- 1 orange, peeled and segmented
- 1/2 grapefruit, peeled and segmented
- 1/2 cup Greek yogurt
- 1 tablespoon honey
- 1/2 cup water
- Ice cubes (optional)

Instructions:

1. Blend orange segments, grapefruit segments, Greek yogurt, and honey.

2. Add water and blend until smooth.

3. Introduce ice cubes if desired, blend again, and revel in the burst of citrus flavors.

Nutrition Information:

- Calories: 160
- Protein: 6g
- Carbohydrates: 30g
- Fat: 2g
- Fiber: 4g
- Sugar: 22g
- Portion Size: 1 serving

Blueberry and Oat Smoothie

Ingredients:

- 1 cup blueberries
- 1/2 cup rolled oats
- 1/2 banana
- 1 cup almond milk

- 1 tablespoon honey

- Ice cubes (optional)

Instructions:

1. Blend blueberries, rolled oats, banana, and almond milk until smooth.

2. Add honey and blend again until well combined.

3. Include ice cubes if desired, blend once more, and relish the blueberry-infused goodness.

Nutrition Information:

- Calories: 190

- Protein: 5g

- Carbohydrates: 35g

- Fat: 4g

- Fiber: 6g

- Sugar: 15g

- Portion Size: 1 serving

Chocolate Peanut Butter Protein Smoothie

Ingredients:

- 1 scoop chocolate protein powder
- 2 tablespoons peanut butter
- 1 banana
- 1 cup milk (dairy or plant-based)
- 1 tablespoon chia seeds
- Ice cubes (optional)

Instructions:

1. Blend chocolate protein powder, peanut butter, banana, and milk until creamy.
2. Add chia seeds and blend until well incorporated.
3. Introduce ice cubes if desired, blend once more, and indulge in the protein-packed delight.

Nutrition Information:

- Calories: 280
- Protein: 20g
- Carbohydrates: 25g
- Fat: 12g

- Fiber: 5g

- Sugar: 15g

- Portion Size: 1 serving

Cucumber and Mint Cooler Smoothie

Ingredients:

- 1 cucumber, peeled and sliced

- 1/2 cup fresh mint leaves

- 1/2 lime, juiced

- 1 tablespoon honey

- 1 cup coconut water

- Ice cubes (optional)

Instructions:

1. Blend cucumber slices, fresh mint leaves, lime juice, and honey until smooth.

2. Add coconut water and blend until well mixed.

3. Include ice cubes if desired, blend again, and relish the cooling sensation.

Nutrition Information:

- Calories: 100

- Protein: 2g
- Carbohydrates: 25g
- Fat: 0g
- Fiber: 3g
- Sugar: 15g
- Portion Size: 1 serving

Peach and Ginger Smoothie

Ingredients:

- 1 cup sliced peaches
- 1/2 inch fresh ginger, peeled
- 1/2 banana
- 1/2 cup orange juice
- 1/2 cup Greek yogurt
- Ice cubes (optional)

Instructions:

1. Blend sliced peaches, fresh ginger, banana, and orange juice until smooth.
2. Add Greek yogurt and blend until creamy.
3. Introduce ice cubes if desired, blend once more, and savor the peachy delight.

Nutrition Information:

- Calories: 150
- Protein: 4g
- Carbohydrates: 30g
- Fat: 2g
- Fiber: 4g
- Sugar: 20g
- Portion Size: 1 serving

Kiwi and Lime Smoothie

Ingredients:

- 2 kiwis, peeled and sliced
- 1/2 lime, juiced
- 1/2 cup pineapple chunks
- 1 tablespoon honey
- 1 cup coconut water
- Ice cubes (optional)

Instructions:

1. Blend kiwi slices, lime juice, pineapple chunks, and honey until smooth.
2. Add coconut water and blend until well combined.

3. Include ice cubes if desired, blend again, and enjoy the tropical fusion.

Nutrition Information:

- Calories: 130
- Protein: 2g
- Carbohydrates: 30g
- Fat: 1g
- Fiber: 5g
- Sugar: 20g
- Portion Size: 1 serving

Papaya and Orange Smoothie

Ingredients:

- 1 cup papaya chunks
- 1 orange, peeled and segmented
- 1/2 banana
- 1/2 cup Greek yogurt
- 1 tablespoon flaxseeds
- Ice cubes (optional)

Instructions:

1. Blend papaya chunks, orange segments, banana, and Greek yogurt until smooth.

2. Add flaxseeds and blend until well mixed.

3. Introduce ice cubes if desired, blend once more, and delight in the tropical fusion.

Nutrition Information:

- Calories: 160
- Protein: 5g
- Carbohydrates: 30g
- Fat: 3g
- Fiber: 6g
- Sugar: 20g
- Portion Size: 1 serving

Beetroot and Berry Smoothie

Ingredients:

- 1/2 cup cooked beetroot, diced
- 1 cup mixed berries (strawberries, blueberries, raspberries)
- 1/2 cup coconut water

- 1 tablespoon honey

- 1/2 cup Greek yogurt

- Ice cubes (optional)

Instructions:

1. Blend cooked beetroot, mixed berries, coconut water, and honey until smooth.

2. Add Greek yogurt and blend until creamy.

3. Include ice cubes if desired, blend again, and enjoy the vibrant, nutrient-packed smoothie.

Nutrition Information:

- Calories: 180

- Protein: 6g

- Carbohydrates: 35g

- Fat: 2g

- Fiber: 8g

- Sugar: 20g

- Portion Size: 1 serving

Turmeric and Pineapple Smoothie

Ingredients:

- 1 cup pineapple chunks
- 1/2 teaspoon ground turmeric
- 1/2 banana
- 1/2 cup almond milk
- 1 tablespoon chia seeds
- Ice cubes (optional)

Instructions:

1. Blend pineapple chunks, ground turmeric, banana, and almond milk until smooth.
2. Add chia seeds and blend until well combined.
3. Introduce ice cubes if desired, blend once more, and relish the anti-inflammatory goodness.

Nutrition Information:

- Calories: 150
- Protein: 4g
- Carbohydrates: 30g
- Fat: 5g
- Fiber: 6g

- Sugar: 18g
- Portion Size: 1 serving

CONCLUSION

The Vegetarian Type 2 Diabetes Cookbook for Beginners" is more than just a collection of recipes; it's a guide to transforming your relationship with food and managing diabetes through delicious, wholesome meals. Throughout the journey from the introductory chapters to the concluding pages, we've embarked on a flavorful exploration of plant-based nutrition tailored to those navigating the challenges of Type 2 Diabetes.

The 30-day meal plan provides a structured approach, ensuring not only variety in your diet but also a well-balanced intake of nutrients. Each section, whether it be the energizing breakfasts, satisfying lunches, hearty dinners, enticing snacks, guilt-free desserts, or refreshing smoothies, serves a purpose beyond satiating your taste buds. It's a roadmap to maintaining blood sugar levels, promoting overall health, and enjoying food in a way that aligns with your dietary preferences and health goals.

Beyond the recipes, this cookbook is a celebration of the potential within plant-based ingredients to create culinary masterpieces. From the simplicity of a quinoa salad to the richness of a chocolate avocado cake, we've showcased the diverse and exciting world of vegetarian cuisine. These recipes not only nourish the body but also awaken the senses, proving that managing diabetes can be a flavorful and enjoyable experience.

As we reach the conclusion of this culinary journey, remember that adopting a vegetarian lifestyle for diabetes management is not just a temporary fix but a sustainable lifestyle change. The knowledge gained from these pages empowers you to make informed choices, create delicious meals, and embrace a healthier future. May this cookbook serve as a constant companion on your path to wellness, offering inspiration and guidance as you navigate the intricacies of a vegetarian diet for Type 2 Diabetes. Here's to a vibrant, delicious, and fulfilling life—one recipe at a time.